Juicing Cleanse and Detoxification

15 Easy Juicing Recipes and Diet

Table of Contents

The Juicing Diet

The juicing diet is a temporary diet that is used to cleanse the body from toxins. It's also used to heal your body with nutrient dense fruits and vegetables and antioxidants. This diet can also be used for weight loss and to reset your body.

If you're interested in trying something new, resetting your body, detoxification, and achieving some weight loss, then this is a diet that you might want to consider.

Now, in order to achieve beneficial results from this diet, you'll need to follow the steps that I list below.

<u>**Juicing Plan**</u>

<u>*3 Days Before the Cleanse:*</u>

Prepare your body with a low inflammatory diet before you start your cleanse. Basically, you'll need to eat a clean diet.

Try to incorporate:

- Dark vegetables
- Fruits besides mangos and bananas
- Grains like quinoa, brown rice, amaranth, and millet
- Beans, legumes and lentils
- Nuts and seeds
- Eggs, chicken, and fish
- Probiotic drinks like kombucha and coconut water.
- Keep hydrated by drinking about 8 to 12 glasses daily.
- If you need caffeine then drink green tea.

Avoid everything else

<u>*Cleansing*</u>

During:

- Start each morning with a warm glass of water with lemon.
- Sip a new juice every 2 hours during the day.
- If you can, try to steam your body or take nightly baths with Epsom salts and lavender essential oils.
- If you get hungry during the cleanse, then stick to fruits, vegetables, and soaked nuts.
- Limit your exercise to light walks.

Even though it's not incorporated into the juice recipes, it's a good idea to add a plant-based protein fiber powder to at 1-2 of your juices per day

3 Days after Cleansing

This is the time when you want to ease your body back into consuming solid foods.

Day 1: Fruits, vegetables, green juices, herbs, green smoothies, and nuts/seeds.

Day 2: Add salads, soups, and heavier protein smoothies.

Day 3: Add clean proteins and gluten-free grains.

When it comes to exercising, you need to listen to your body and know your limits.

Below is a list of juice cleansing recipes that you can choose from. Please enjoy!

If you're a vegan and are interested in some foods that you can eat on the third day after the cleanse, then feel free to check out my book: "_The Vegan's Cookbook_"

https://www.amazon.com/Vegans-Cookbook-Delicious-Vegetarian-Plant-Based-ebook/dp/B074L8HKN8/ref=sr_1_1?ie=UTF8&qid=1502592062&sr=8-1&keywords=amber+swaney

Vegetables and Fruits

Apple	Apples are a good source of soluble fiber and immune boosting vitamin C. Apples help to aid in weight loss and has been shown to lower cholesterol and heart disease markers. Also, apples help to protect against metabolic syndrome, and it can boost exercise endurance as well.
Beets	Beets have been known to lower your blood pressure and boost your stamina. They also fight inflammation, have anti-cancer properties, and help detoxify your body by purifying your blood and liver. Also, beets are rich in valuable nutrients, like vitamin C, vitamin B, manganese, potassium, and fiber.
Cabbage (Red)	Red cabbage helps to aid in weight loss, boost the immune system, and prevent the risk of lung and breast cancer. It also helps to prevent cataracts and macular degeneration. Cabbage protects against Alzheimer's disease and reduces the signs of aging.
Carrots	Carrots have been known to help prevent heart diseases, improve eyesight, and boost the immune system. They also help to regulate blood sugar levels, reduce high blood pressure, and maintain good digestive health. Also, carrots help to prevent macular degeneration and reduce the risk of cancer and stroke.
Celery	Celery is used to manage diabetic symptoms, relieves migraine and asthma, and reduces blood pressure and cholesterol. Celery also prevents urinary tract infections, helps to reduce pain and swelling around the joints. Also, celery promotes cardiovascular health, and prevents cancer and improves immunity. Finally, this vegetable helps to improve eyesight and prevents macular degeneration.
Cucumbers	Cucumbers help to prevent constipation, aid in weight loss, lower blood pressure, and aids in managing diabetes. Also, cucumbers reduce the risk of kidney stones, keep the body healthy, flushes out toxins, and provide a glowing complexion.

Dandelion Greens	Dandelion greens provide an enormous amount of vitamin K, vitamin A, and a flavoid called zeaxanthin, which protects the retina from UV rays. These greens are also high in fiber, contain vitamin C and B6, thiamin, riboflavin, calcium, and iron. Also, these greens contain potassium, manganese, folate, magnesium, phosphorus, and copper.
Ginger	Ginger has been known to reduce pain and inflammation and gives a warming effect which helps with circulation. Also, it inhibits rhinovirus, which causes the common cold. This plant reduces gas and painful spasms, and inhibits bacteria that cause diarrhea and protozoa.
Grapefruit	Grapefruits help to decrease appetite, prevent acid formation, and promote sleep. It also treats malaria and fatigue, boosts the immune system, and is a valuable remedy for influenza. Also, grapefruit solves problems of indigestion, and regulates sugar levels in diabetics.
Kale	Kale is known for its anti-inflammatory properties, abundance of antioxidants, heart support, and healthy vision. It's also known for its detoxification properties, brain development in infants, and cancer prevention.
Lemon	Lemons help to reduce weight, control high blood pressure, stops internal bleeding, and treat arthritis. Lemons also provide relaxation to the feet, gives relief from fever, soothes toothache, and eases the pain of sunburn. Also, lemons cure indigestion, constipation, dandruff, and help to fade scars, remove wrinkles, and blackheads.
Limes	Limes help to stimulate the digestive system, rejuvenate and protect the skin from infection. It also regulates sugar absorption, aids in weight loss, and gives relief from eye infections, arthritis, nausea, gout, and fever. Limes also help to cure scurvy and eliminate dandruff.
Mandarins	Mandarin oranges help with cancer prevention, and are a rich source of vitamin C. They help to lower cholesterol and blood pressure. These oranges also aid in weight loss, promote skin

	health, and boost the immune system
Oranges	Oranges are known to boost the immune system, reduce cardiovascular diseases, reduce risk of macular, and protects against cancer. Oranges also improve blood circulation and are rich in antioxidants and anti-inflammatory properties.
Pears	Pears help to boost the immune system, treat eczema and dermatitis, and prevent cancer and cardiovascular diseases. Pears also improve digestion, speeds up the wound healing process, and improve blood circulation.
Pineapple	Pineapples help to improve oral and eye health, boost the immune system and blood circulation, and reduce inflammation of the joints and muscles. Pineapples also help to heal wounds, prevent arthritis, cancer, and heart diseases, reduce the risk of dementia and Alzheimer's disease, and protects against constipation.
Romaine Lettuce	Romaine lettuce has a good amount of B vitamins, vitamin A, vitamin C, and vitamin K. It also has omega-3 fatty acids, dietary fiber, molybdenum, and minerals like iron, potassium, calcium, copper, magnesium, chromium, manganese, and phosphorus.
Spinach	Spinach is known for improving eyesight, aids in strengthening muscles, prevents osteoporosis, boosts metabolism, and help maintain normal blood pressure. Spinach also helps to provide the body with neurological benefits, and prevents macular degeneration.
Sweet Potato	Sweet potatoes provide relief from arthritis, boosts the immune system, helps to treat cancer, and cure stomach ulcers. They also maintain water balance within the body and are excellent for digestion.
Turmeric Root	Turmeric is used to help with pain relief, depression, and contains anti-inflammatory properties. It also helps with skin conditions, cancer, arthritis, weight loss, diabetes, cholesterol, and digestion.

Beauty Juice

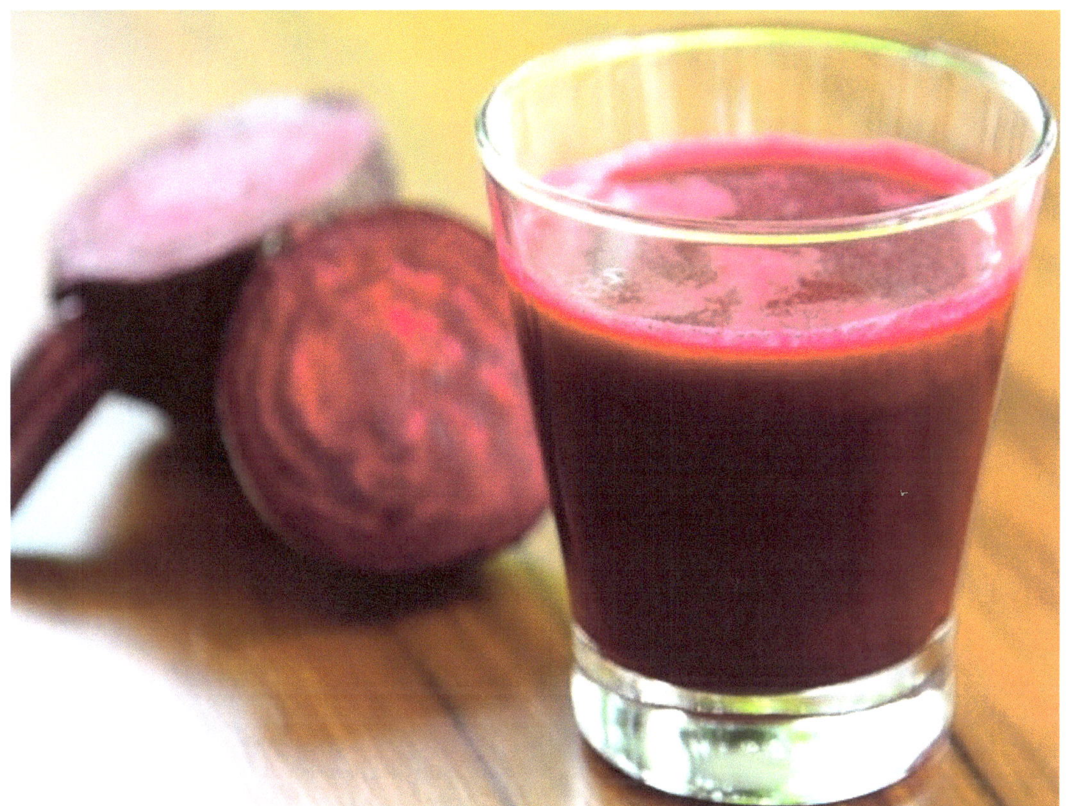

Ingredients:

2 Beets

3 Carrots

1 Lemon

1 Apple

5 Kale Leaves

4 Stalks Celery

1 Inch Ginger

The Cleanser Juice

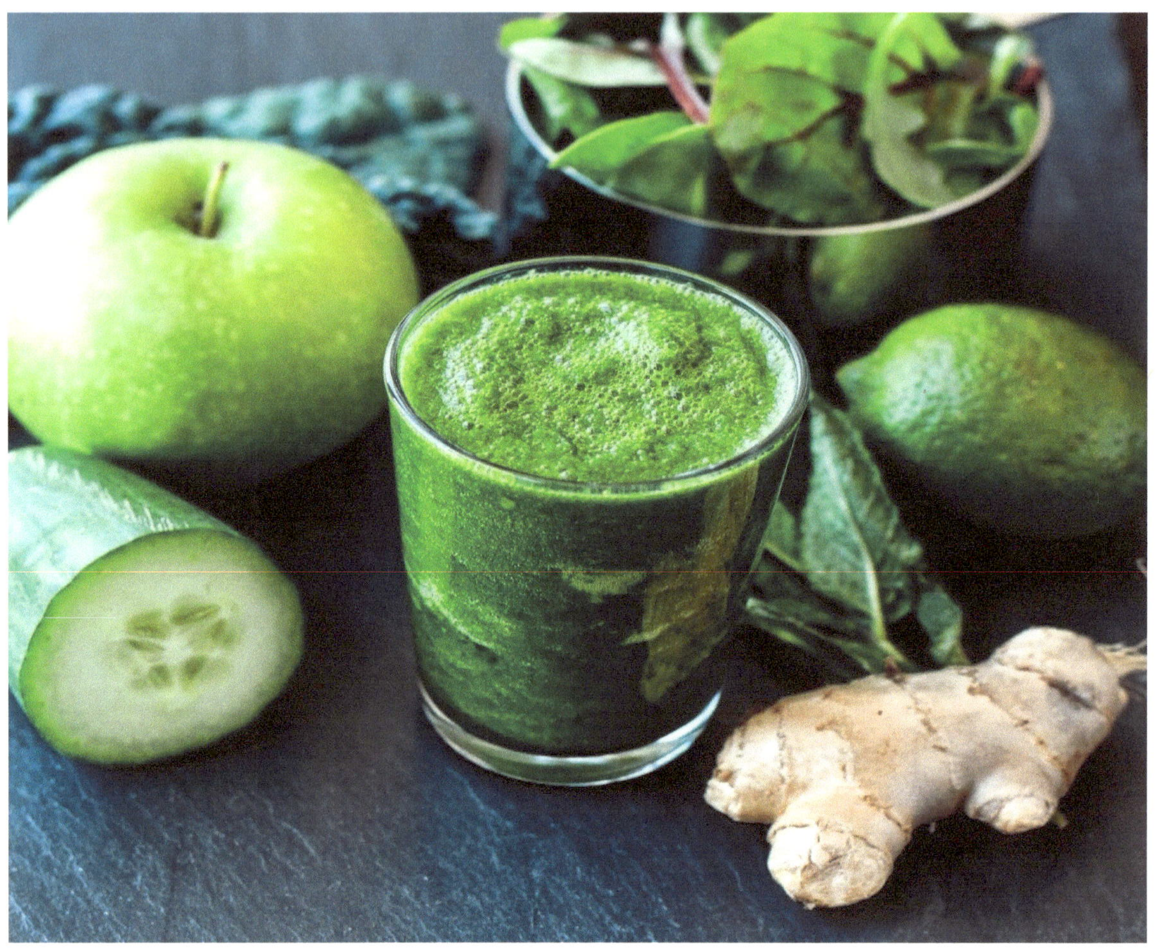

Ingredients

3 Cucumbers, Peeled

3 Organic Hearts of Romaine Lettuce

2 Organic Gala Apples, Cored

1 Organic Celery Heart

½ Lemon

The Cellulite Blaster

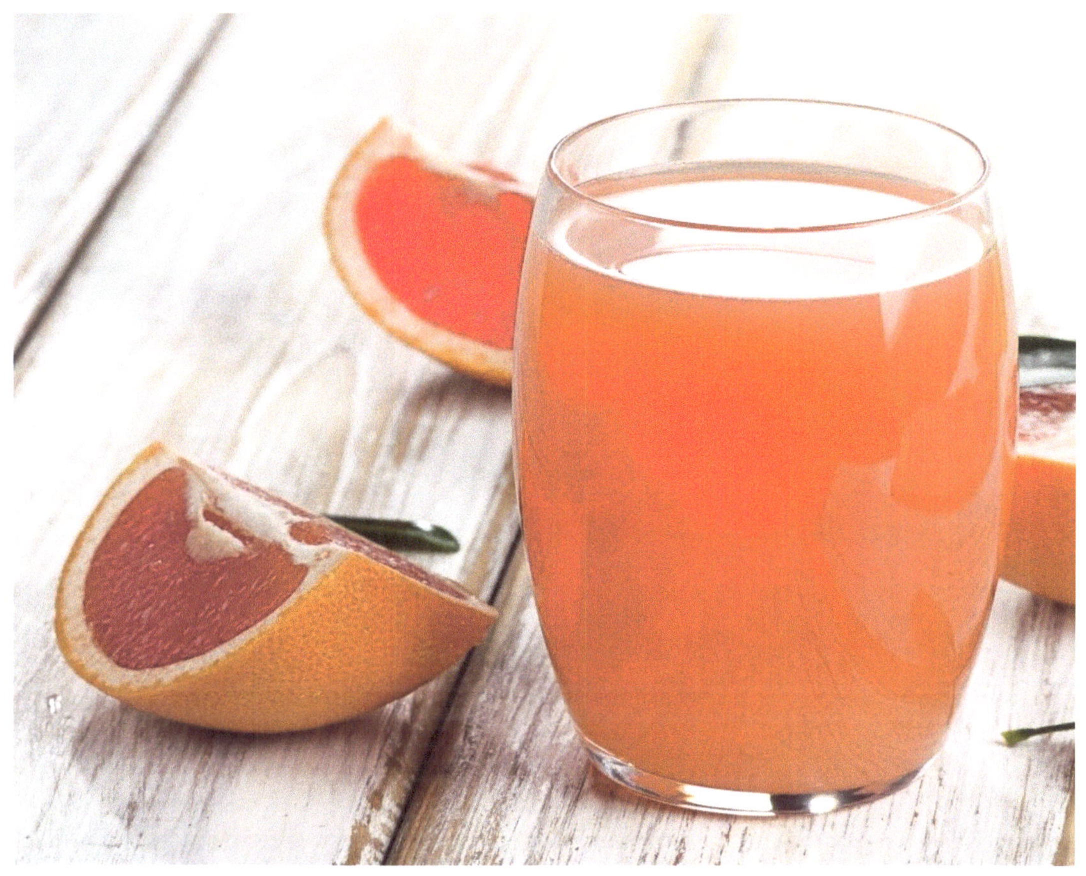

Ingredients

5 Grapefruits

1 Lemon

2 Limes

1/4 Medium Pineapple

Handful of Ginger, you be the judge on how much to use

Green Detox

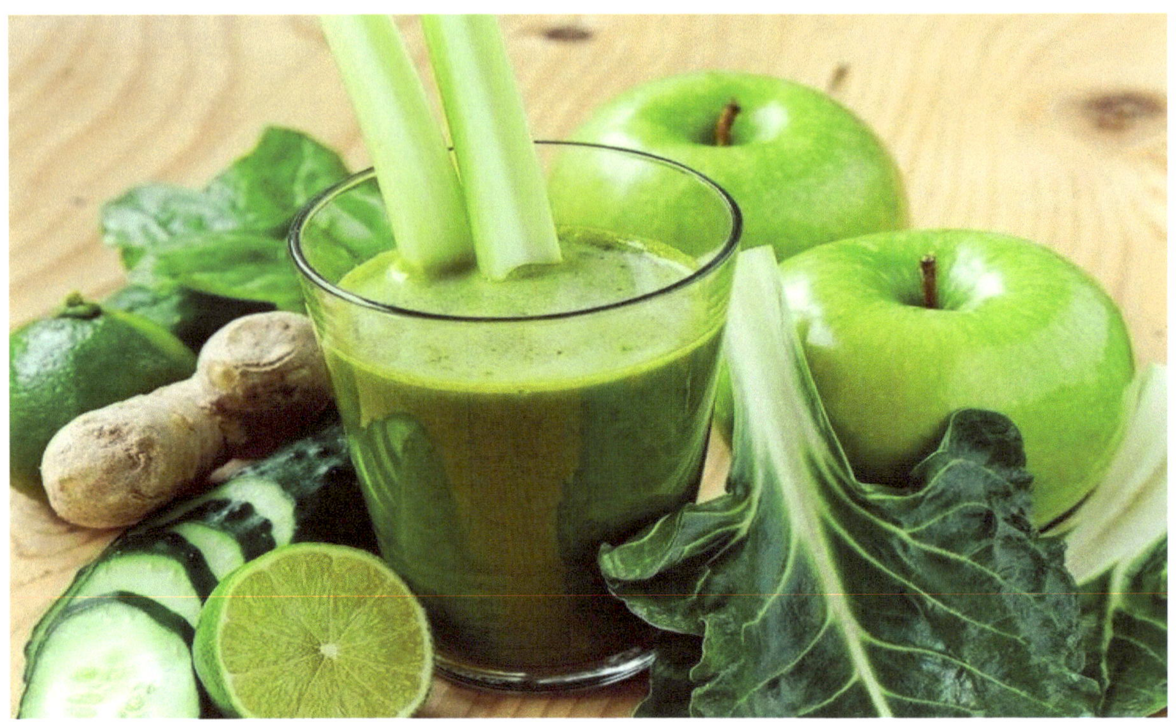

<u>Ingredients</u>

2 Medium Apples

4 Celery

1 Cucumber

1 Inch Ginger Root

6 Kale Leaves

½ Lemon

Green Belly Buster Juice

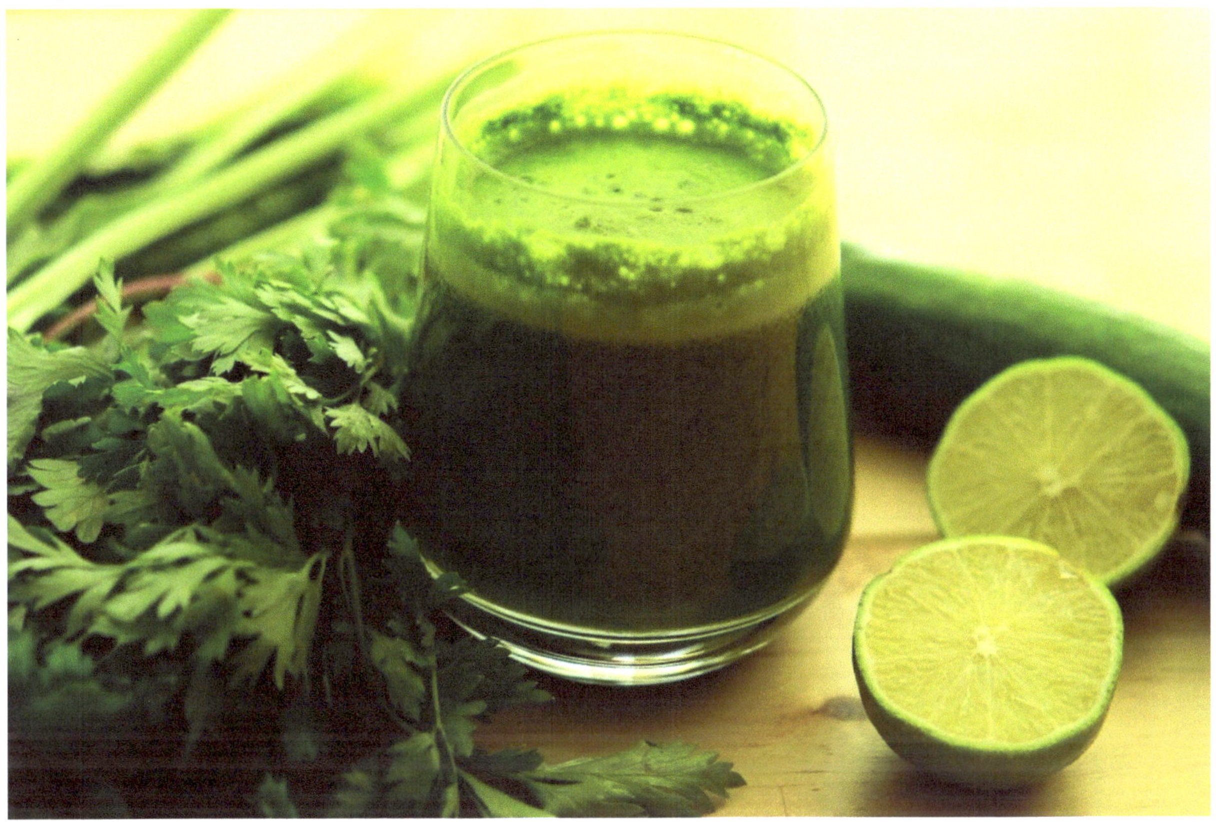

<u>Ingredients</u>

3 Medium Apples

1 Large Cucumber

1 Large Lemon, Including Skin

1 Lime, Including Skin

3 Small Mandarins, Including Skin

1 Head Romaine Lettuce

Beets and Spinach Detox

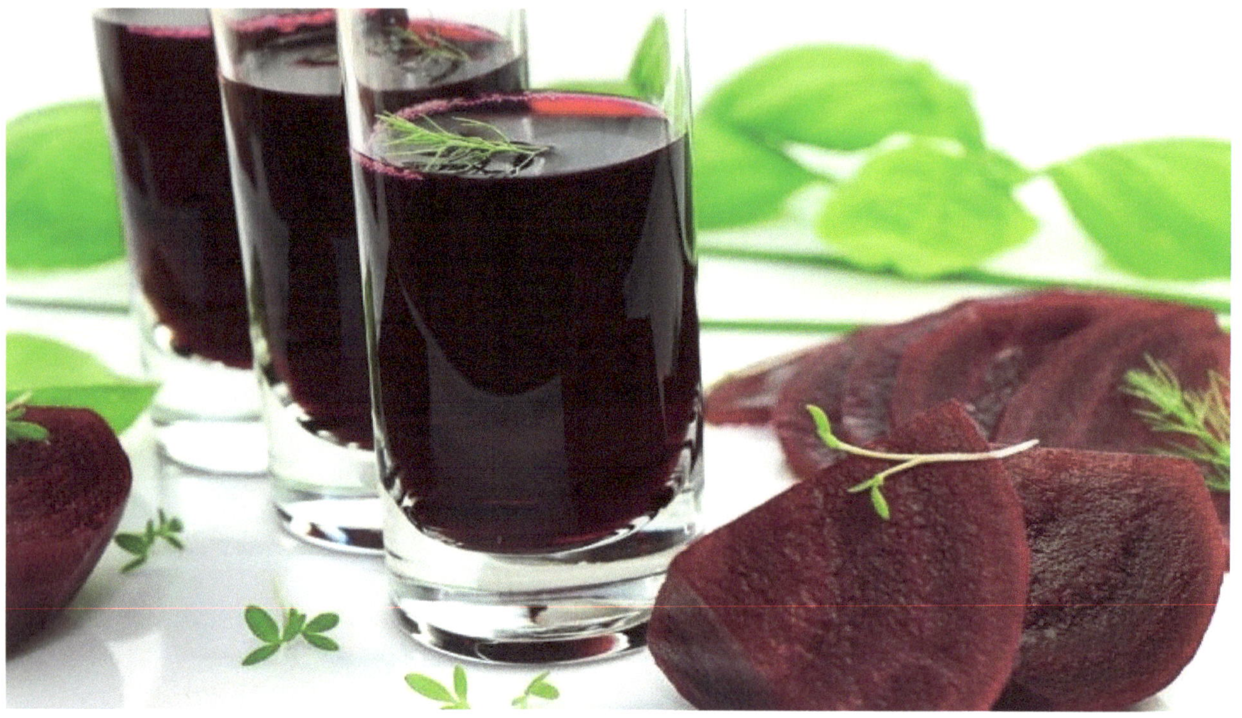

Ingredients

1 Beet Root

2 Cabbage (red) Leaves

3 Medium Carrots

½ Lemon

1 Orange

½ Fruit Pineapple

 2 Handfuls Spinach

Green Lemonade Juice

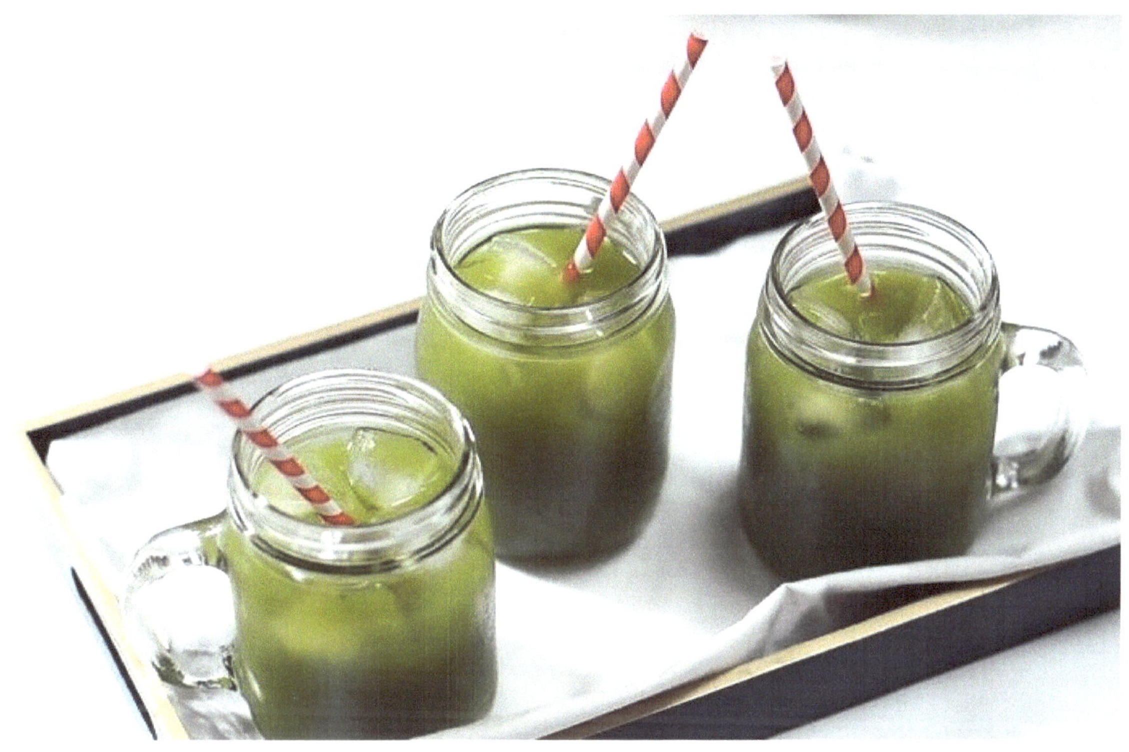

<u>Ingredients</u>

2 Medium Apples

1 Cucumber

4 Kale Leaves

1 Lemon

2 Cups Spinach

Sunset Juice

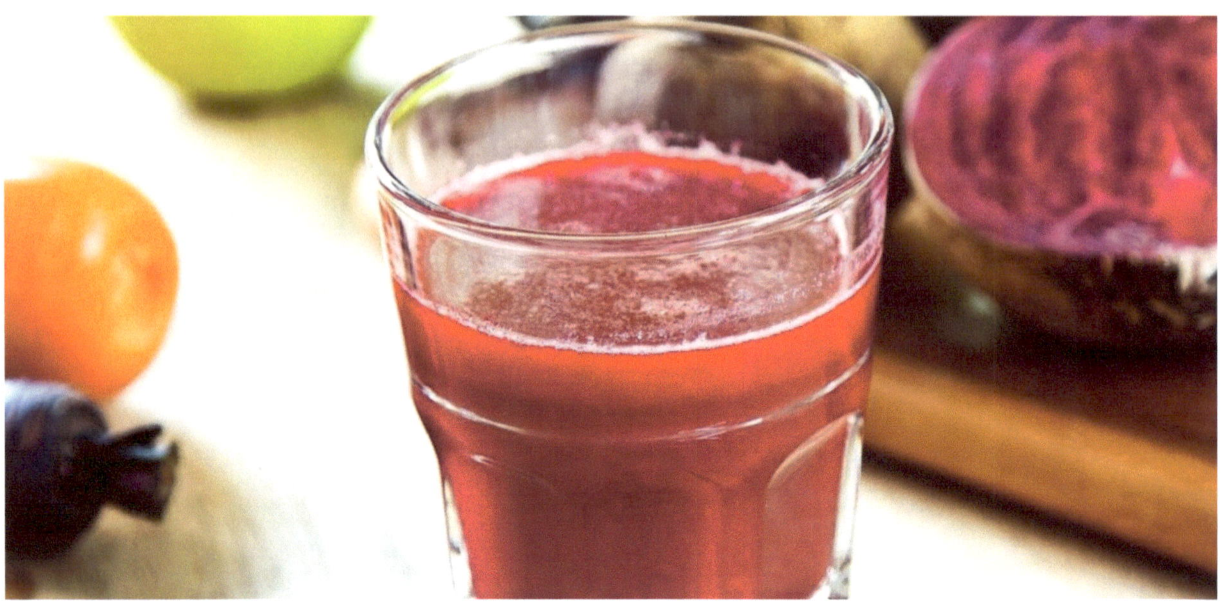

Ingredients

2 Medium Apples

1 Beet Root

1 Large Carrot

1 Orange

1 Sweet Potato

Turmeric Detox

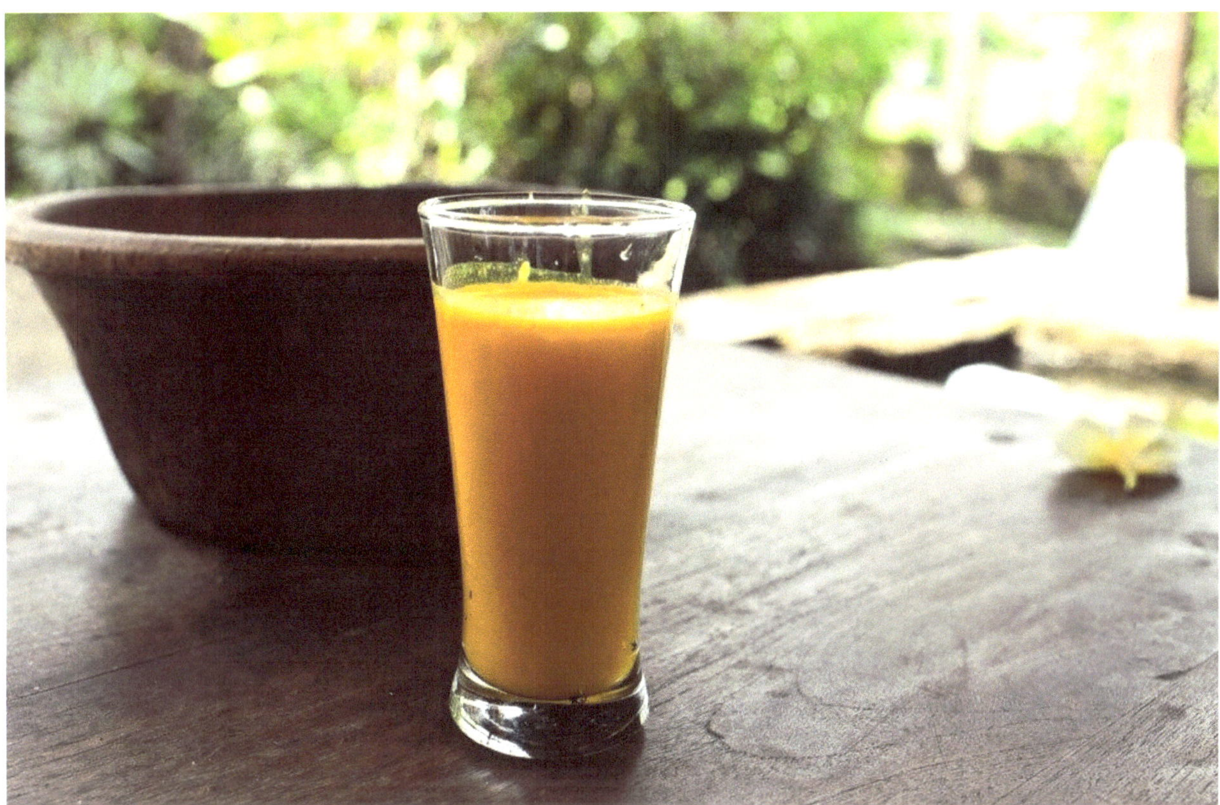

<u>Ingredients</u>

2 Medium Apples

3 Medium Carrots

3 Stalks Celery

1 Ginger Root

2 Lemons (peeled)

2 Medium Pears

6 Turmeric Roots

Workout Juice

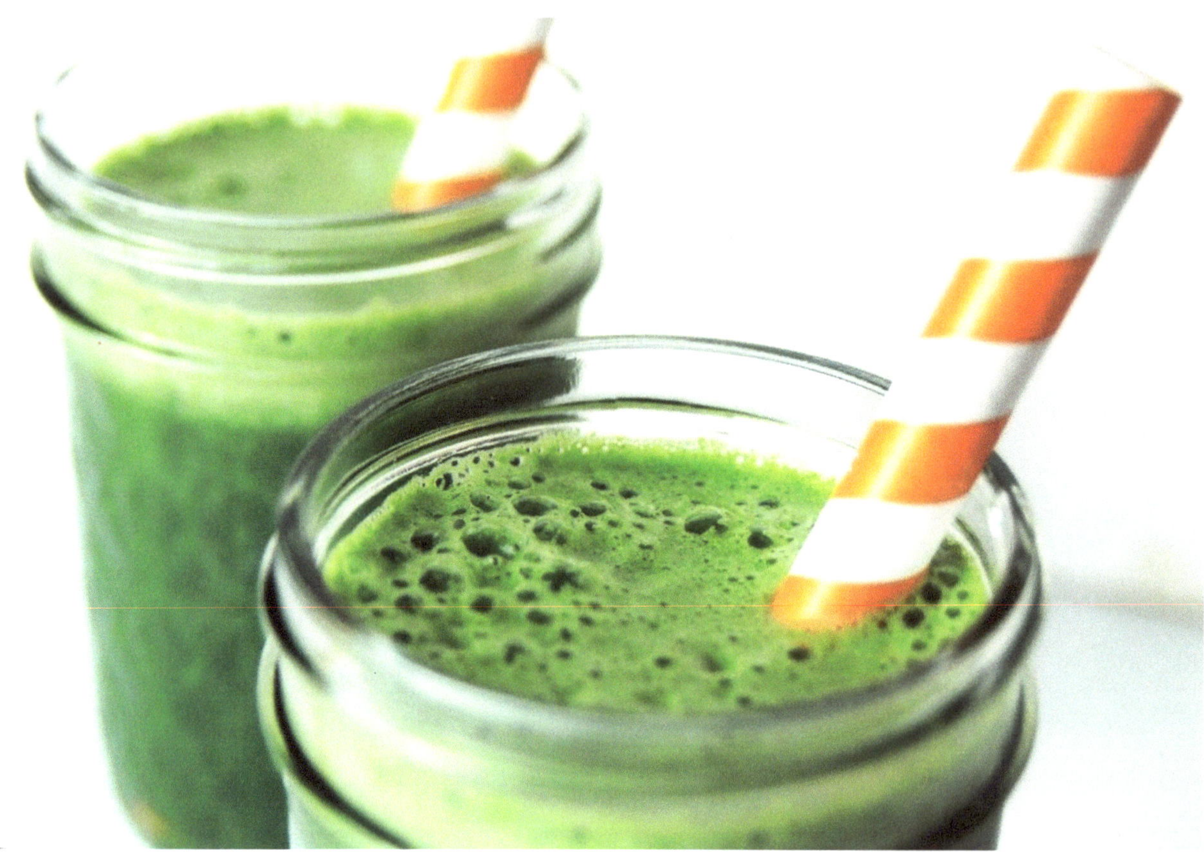

Ingredients

2 Medium Apples

2 Stalks Celery

½ Cucumber

1 Cup Dandelion Greens

3 Kale Leaves

½ Lemon

Mojito Juice

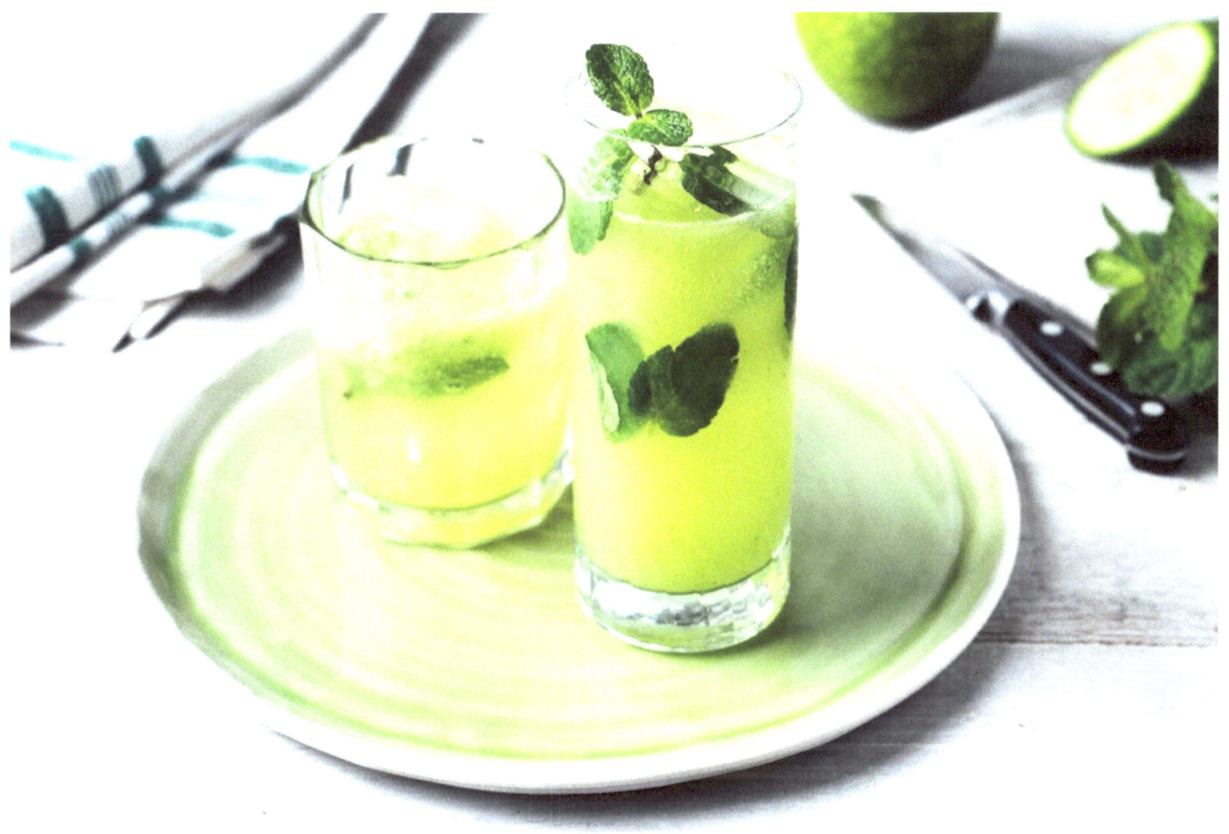

<u>**Ingredients**</u>

1 Cucumber

1 Large Pear

1 Large Handful Mint

½ Lime

Sour and Sweet Detox Juice

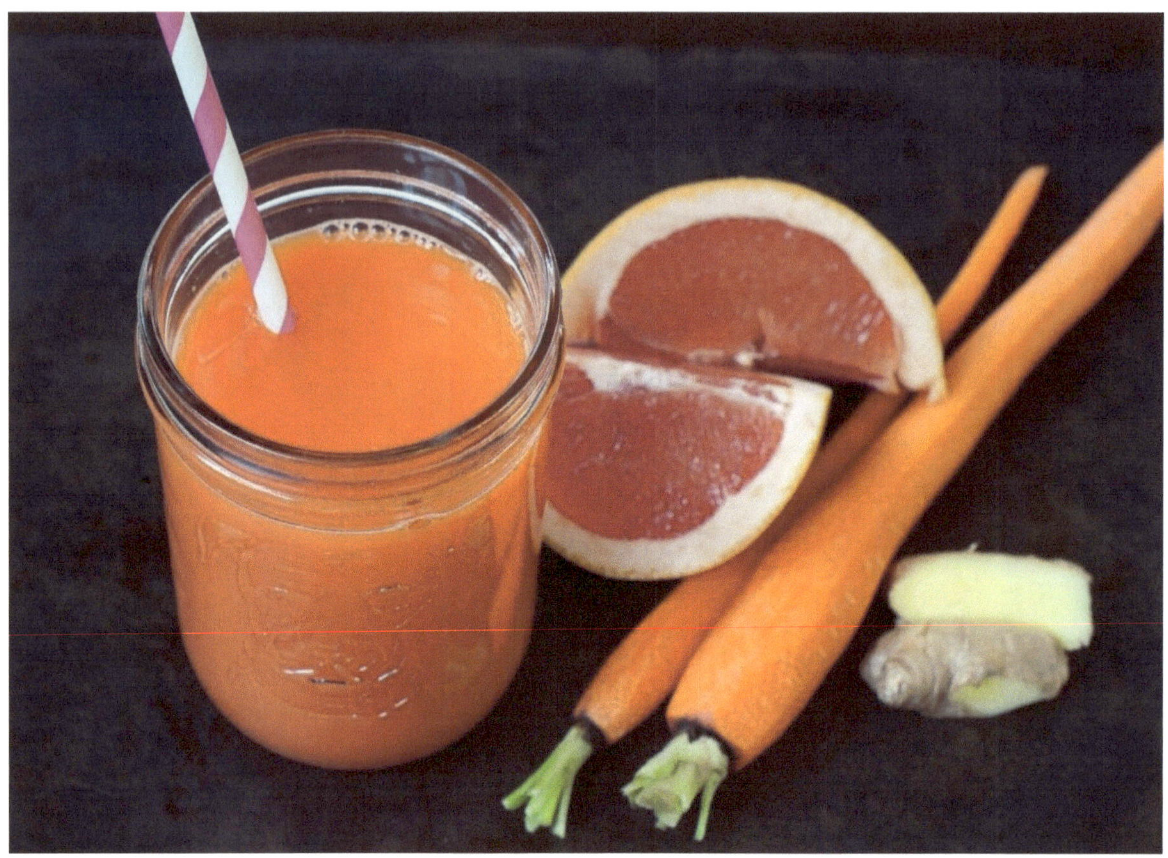

<u>Ingredients</u>

1 Apple

4 Large Carrots

1 Beet

1 Inch Ginger

1-2 Cups Grapefruit

Pink Cleanse

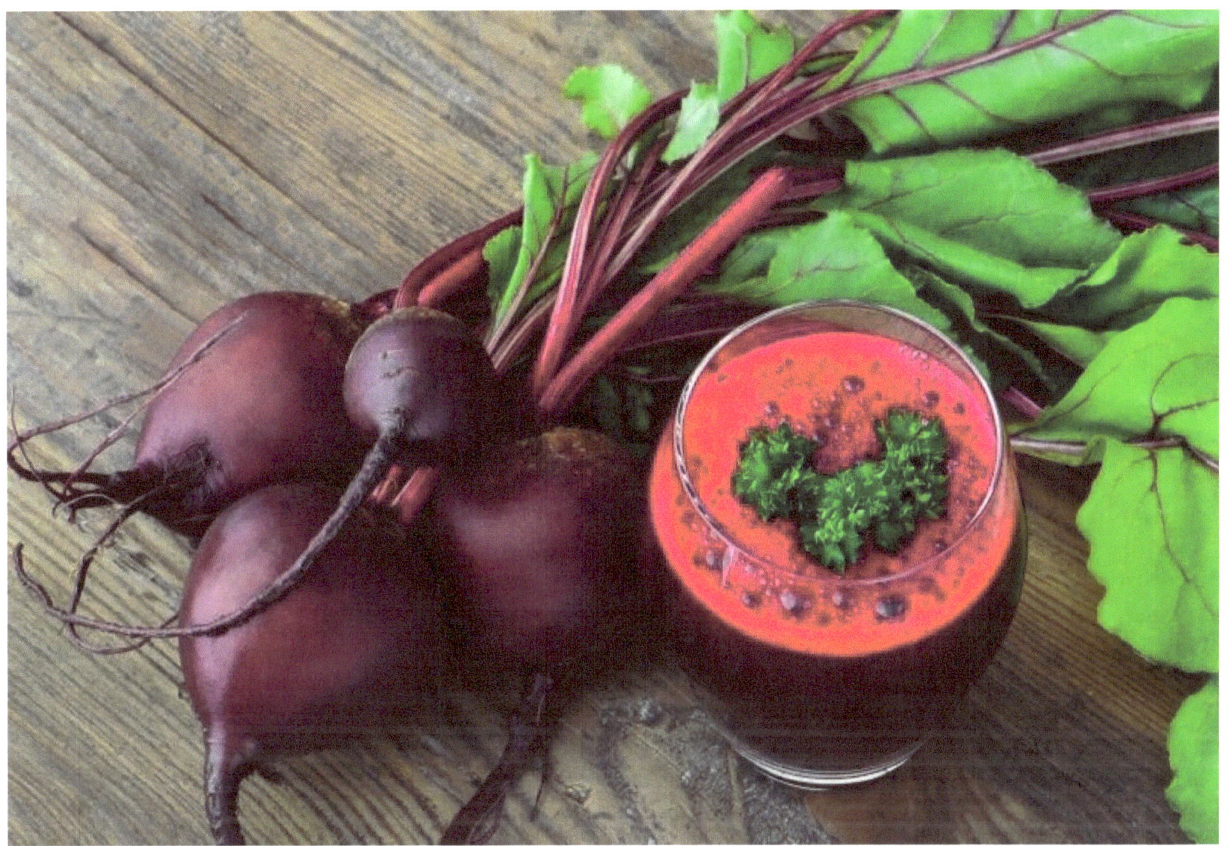

Ingredients

1 Beet

1 Green Apple

1 Pear

6 Romaine Leaves

1 Inch Ginger

Carrot Apple Detox

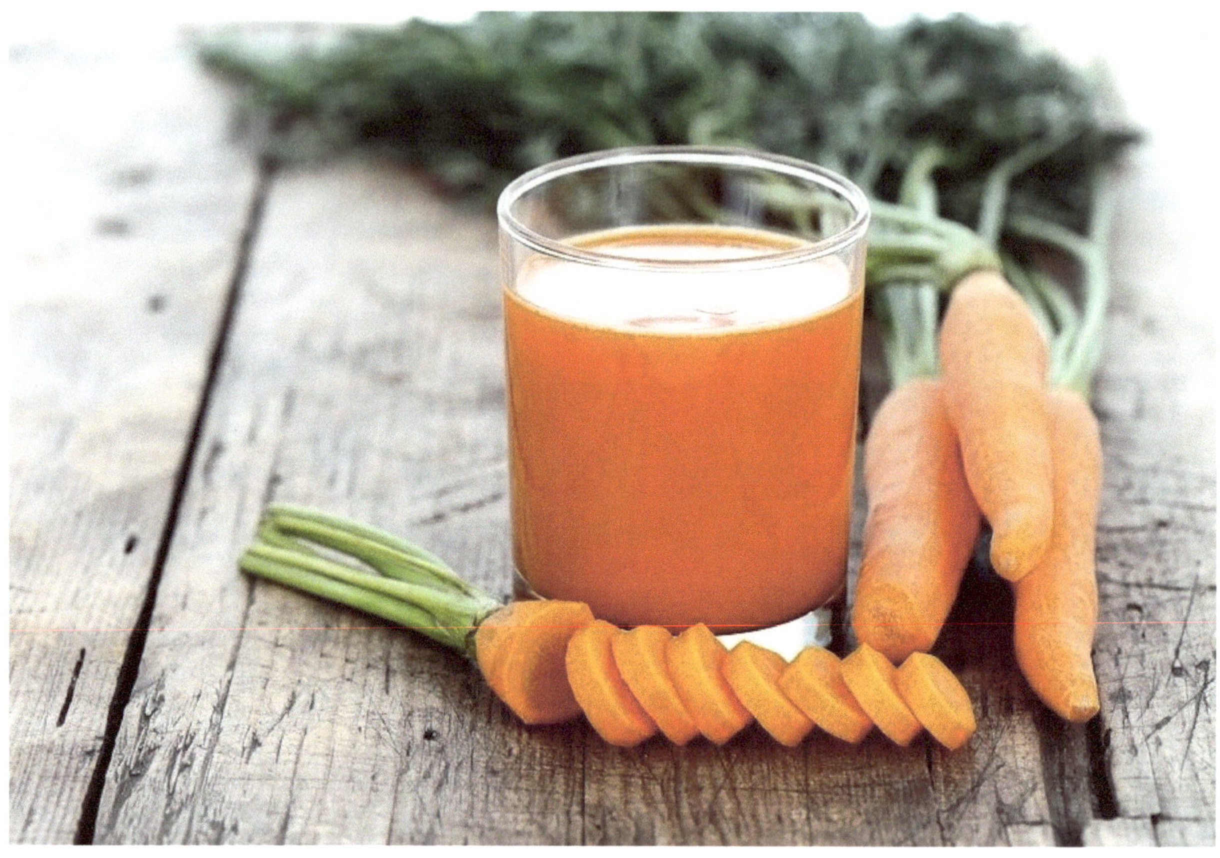

Ingredients

1 Large Apple, Quartered

1/4 (15 ounce) Can Pineapple Chunks

2 Large Carrots

2 Pieces Fresh Ginger

Lemon Apple Juice Cleanse

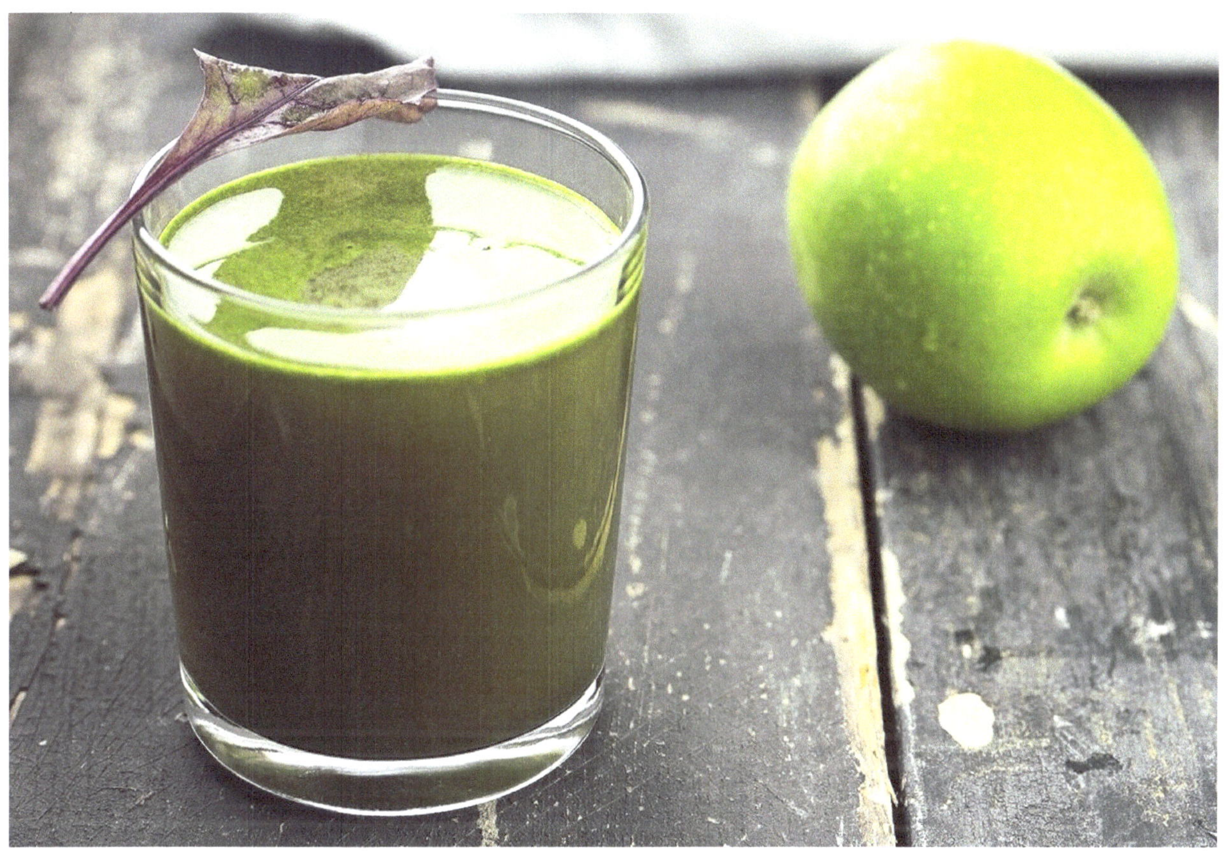

Ingredients

2 Lemons, Peeled and Halved

4 Apples, Quartered

2 Cucumbers, Halved

1 Cup Water

Conclusion

Thank you for ordering and/or downloading my book. I hope you enjoyed it and it had positive effects on you.

Juicing can be a great way to cleanse the body of toxins and to reset your diet. It helps to rejuvenate the body, leaving you feeling like a new, healthier person.

Please a leave a review if you can, and thank you again!

Work Cited

"10 Amazing Health Benefits of Eating Celery | Food and Nutrition." *Daily Free Health Articles and Natural Health Advice*, 22 Apr. 2016, www.doctorshealthpress.com/food-and-nutrition-articles/10-health-benefits-of-celery/.

"10 Impressive Benefits of Carrots." *Organic Facts*, 20 June 2017, www.organicfacts.net/health-benefits/vegetable/carrots.html.

"10 Science-Based Benefits of Grapefruit." *Healthline*, Healthline Media, 18 Feb. 2017, www.healthline.com/nutrition/10-benefits-of-grapefruit.

"16 Health Benefits of Lemons." *16 Health Benefits Of Lemons | Care2 Healthy Living*, www.care2.com/greenliving/16-health-benefits-of-lemons.html.

"16 Superb Health Benefits of Cucumber." *16 Superb Health Benefits Of Cucumber | Care2 Healthy Living*, www.care2.com/greenliving/16-superb-health-benefits-of-cucumber.html.

"5 Health Benefits of an Apple." *EatingWell*, EatingWell, 20 Sept. 2011, www.eatingwell.com/article/17769/5-health-benefits-of-an-apple/.

"9 Health Benefits of Sweet Potatoes." *9 Health Benefits Of Sweet Potatoes | Care2 Healthy Living*, www.care2.com/greenliving/9-reasons-to-love-sweet-potatoes.html.

"9 Impressive Benefits of Red Cabbage." *Organic Facts*, 28 June 2017, www.organicfacts.net/health-benefits/vegetable/red-cabbage.html.

"Six Amazing Health Benefits of Eating Beets." *Mercola.com*, http://articles.mercola.com/sites/articles/archive/2014/01/25/beets-health-benefits.aspx.

"What Are Dandelion Greens Good For?" *Mercola.com*, http://foodfacts.mercola.com/dandelion-greens.html.

"What Is Romaine Lettuce Good For?" *Mercola.com*, http://foodfacts.mercola.com/romaine-lettuce.html.

"What Is Spinach Good For?" *Mercola.com*, http://foodfacts.mercola.com/spinach.html.

Akruti. "14 Amazing Benefits Of Mandarin Oranges For Skin, Hair and Health." *STYLECRAZE*, IncnutIncnut, www.stylecraze.com/articles/benefits-of-mandarin-oranges-for-skin-hair-and-health/#gref.

Boldt, Ethan. "Health Benefits of Kale + Kale Nutrition & Kale Recipes." *Dr. Axe*, 5 July 2017, http://draxe.com/health-benefits-of-kale/.

Dr. Josh Axe and Eric Zielinski. "Turmeric Benefits Superior To 10 Medications At Reversing
Disease." *Dr. Axe*, 3 Aug. 2017, http://draxe.com/turmeric-benefits/.

Fanous, Summer. "8 Healthy Lime Facts." *Healthline*, Healthline Media, 5 May 2016,
www.healthline.com/health/8-healthy-lime-facts.

Oranges, www.whfoods.com/genpage.php?tname=foodspice&dbid=37.

Publications, Inc. Ogden. "5 Health Benefits of Pears - Natural Health." *Mother Earth Living*, 14 Feb.
2012, www.motherearthliving.com/Natural-Health/5-health-benefits-of-pears.

Veronica, et al. "19 Science-Backed Health Benefits of Pineapple." *Well-Being Secrets*, 24 Jan. 2017,
www.well-beingsecrets.com/health-benefits-of-pineapple/.

White, MD Linda B. "7 Health Benefits of Ginger." *The Remedy Chicks*, 23 Dec. 2014,
www.everydayhealth.com/columns/white-seeber-grogan-the-remedy-chicks/health-benefits-
ginger/.